The Ultimate Vegetarian Breakfast Cookbook

Delicious Vegetarian Breakfast
Recipes To Start The Day

Adam Denton

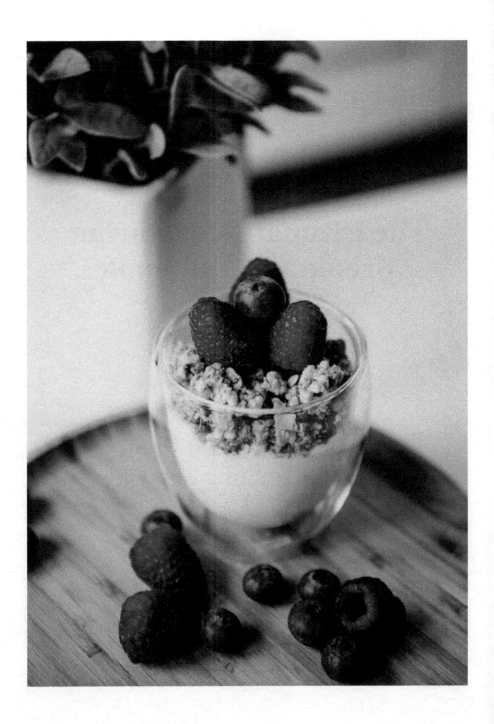

Table of contents

5

Milky Scrambled Tofu

Preparation Time: 10 minutes

Cooking time: 10 minutes

Servings: 4

Ingredients:

7 ounces almond milk

2 tablespoons flax meal mixed with 2 tablespoons water

2 tablespoons firm tofu, crumbled

Cooking spray

Salt and black pepper to the taste

8 cherry tomatoes, cut into halves

Directions:

In a bowl, mix flax meal with milk, salt and pepper and whisk well. Grease your air fryer with cooking spray, pour flax meal, add tofu, cook at 350 degrees F for 6 minutes, scramble them a bit and transfer to plates. Divide tomatoes on top and serve. Enjoy!

Breakfast Bell Peppers

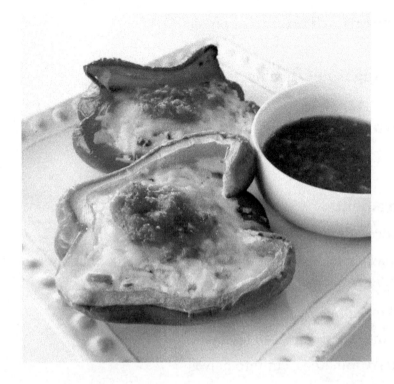

Preparation Time: 10 minutes

Cooking time: 10 minutes

Servings: 8

Ingredients:

1 yellow bell pepper, halved

1 orange bell pepper, halved

Salt and black pepper to the taste

ounces firm tofu, crumbled

1 green onion, chopped

2 tablespoons oregano, chopped

Directions:

In a bowl, mix tofu with onion, salt, pepper and oregano and stir well. Place bell pepper halves in your air fryer's basket and cook at 400 degrees F for 10 minutes. Leave bell pepper halves to cool down, peel, divide tofu mix on each piece, roll, arrange on plates and serve right away for breakfast. Enjoy!

French Toast Pudding

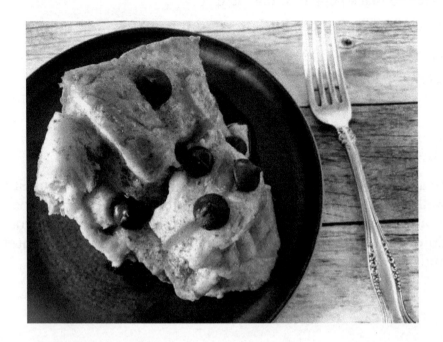

Preparation Time: 5 minutes

Cooking time: 0 minutes

Servings: 5

Ingredients:

4 Bananas, Chopped

1 Cup Almond Milk

2 Tablespoons Maple Syrup

4 Slices Vegan French Bread

1 Teaspoon Vanilla Extract, Pure

1 Tablespoon Almond Butter

¼ Teaspoon Ground Cloves

1 Teaspoon Cinnamon

1 Cup Water

Directions:

Pour in your water, and then get out a round pan. Chop the bread and place it on the bottom. Blend your maple syrup, chopped bananas, vanilla extract, cloves and cinnamon together until smooth, pouring it into the pan with the bread. Cover the pan with foil and make sure the edges are secure. Transfer it into the instant pot and then close your lid. Cook on high for sixteen minutes on the pudding setting. Use a quick release, and then add your almond butter in, and stir gently before serving.

Morning Forest Maple Granola

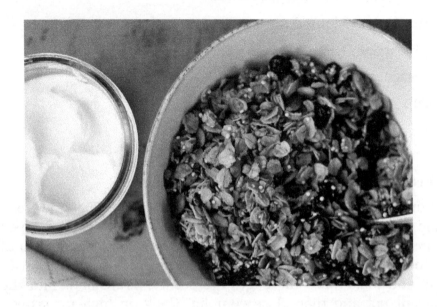

Preparation Time: 5 minutes

Cooking time: 20 minutes

Servings: 4 ½ cups.

Ingredients:

2 cups oats

1/3 cup pumpkin seeds

1/3 cup sunflower seeds

1/3 cup walnuts

1/3 cup unsweetened coconut flakes

¼ cup wheat germ

1 ½ tsp. cinnamon

1 cup raisins

1/3 cup maple syrup

Directions:

Begin by preheating the oven to 325 degrees Fahrenheit. Next, mix all of the above Ingredients—except for the raisins and the maple syrup—together in a large bowl. After you've mixed the Ingredients well, add the maple syrup, and completely coat the other Ingredients. Next, spread out this mixture on a baking sheet and bake the granola for twenty minutes, making sure to stir every four minutes or so. After twenty minutes, add the raisins and bake for an additional five minutes. Remove the baking sheet and allow the granola to cool for forty-five minutes. Enjoy!

Silky Whole Wheat Strawberry Pancakes

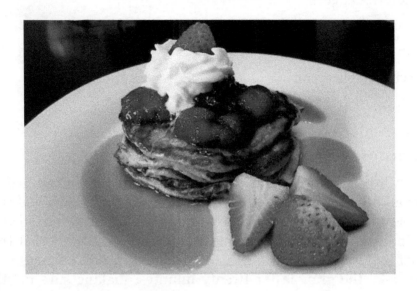

Preparation Time: 5 minutes

Cooking time: 25 minutes

Servings: 24 pancakes.

Ingredients:

1 ¾ cup whole wheat flour

1/3 cup cornmeal

½ tsp. baking soda

1 tsp. baking powder

½ tsp. cinnamon

2 tbsp. maple syrup

2 cups vanilla soymilk

4 cups sliced strawberries

Directions:

Begin by combining all the dry Ingredients together in a mixing bowl. Stir well, and create a hole in the center of the mixture in order to pour the syrup and soymilk into it. Continue to stir, making sure not to over-stir. Next, add half of the strawberries into the mixture. Heat the skillet or the griddle, and portion just a bit of Earth Balance butter overtop. Drop little pieces of the batter onto the skillet and cook both sides of the pancakes. Keep the pancakes warm as you cook the remainder of the batter, and top the pancakes with strawberries. Enjoy.

Whole Wheat Chapatti

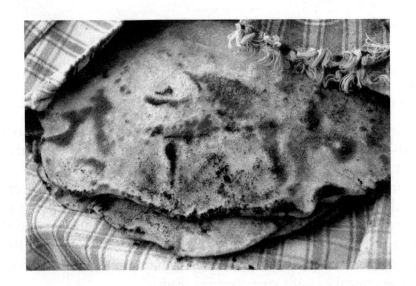

Servings: 8 servings

Preparation Time: 10 mins

Cooking time: 10 mins

Ingredients:

2½ cups whole wheat flour

¾ tsp. salt

1 cup water

Directions:

In a medium-sized bowl, mix together the flour and salt and then stir in water to form a soft, pliable dough. Scrape the dough out onto a lightly floured and clean work surface. Using your hands, knead several times to improve the dough's elasticity and smoothness. Divide the dough into 8 equal portions and roll each into a smooth ball. Using a rolling pin, roll each ball into a very thin circle. Heat a griddle pan over a medium-high heat. Do not add any oil. Cook each dough round on the pan until the dough begins to bubbles and blister, about 2 minutes. Flip over and cook until lightly brown on the other side. Serve immediately.

Hot Pink Smoothie

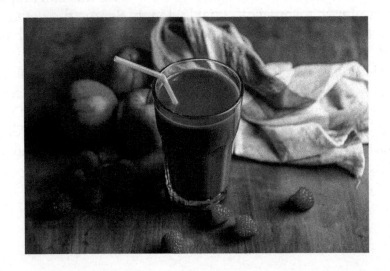

Preparation Time: 5 minutes

Cooking time: 0 minute

Servings: 1

Ingredients:

1 clementine, peeled, segmented

1/2 frozen banana

1 small beet, peeled, chopped

1/8 teaspoon sea salt

1/2 cup raspberries

1 tablespoon chia seeds

¼ teaspoon vanilla extract, unsweetened

2 tablespoons almond butter

1 cup almond milk, unsweetened

Directions:

Place all the Ingredients in the order in a food processor or blender and then pulse for 2 to 3 minutes at high speed until smooth. Pour the smoothie into a glass and then serve.

Chocolate Oat Smoothie

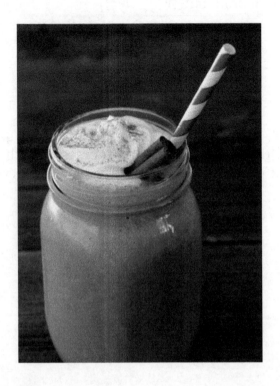

Preparation Time: 5 minutes

Cooking time: 0 minute

Servings: 1

Ingredients:

¼ cup rolled oats

1 ½ tablespoon cocoa powder, unsweetened

1 teaspoon flax seeds

1 large frozen banana

1/8 teaspoon sea salt

1/8 teaspoon cinnamon

¼ teaspoon vanilla extract, unsweetened

2 tablespoons almond butter

1 cup coconut milk, unsweetened

Directions:

Place all the Ingredients in the order in a food processor or blender and then pulse for 2 to 3 minutes at high speed until smooth. Pour the smoothie into a glass and then serve.

Wild Ginger Green Smoothie

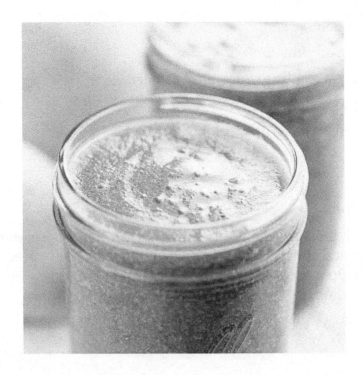

Preparation Time: 5 minutes

Cooking time: 0 minute

Servings: 1

Ingredients:

1/2 cup pineapple chunks, frozen

1/2 cup chopped kale 1/2 frozen banana

1 tablespoon lime juice

2 inches ginger, peeled, chopped

1/2 cup coconut milk, unsweetened

1/2 cup coconut water

Directions:

Place all the Ingredients in the order in a food processor or blender and then pulse for 2 to 3 minutes at high speed until smooth. Pour the smoothie into a glass and then serve

Double Chocolate Hazelnut Espresso Shake

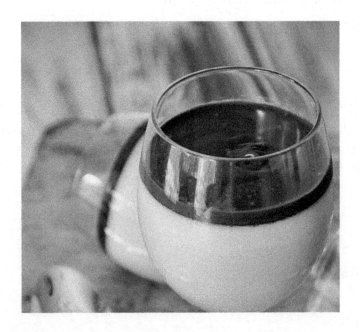

Preparation Time: 5 minutes

Cooking time: 0 minute

Servings: 1

Ingredients:
1 frozen banana, sliced
1/4 cup roasted hazelnuts

4 Medjool dates, pitted, soaked

2 tablespoons cacao nibs, unsweetened

1 1/2 tablespoons cacao powder, unsweetened

1/8 teaspoon sea salt

1 teaspoon vanilla extract, unsweetened

1 cup almond milk, unsweetened

1/2 cup ice

4 ounces espresso, chilled

Directions:

Place all the Ingredients in the order in a food processor or blender and then pulse for 2 to 3 minutes at high speed until smooth. Pour the smoothie into a glass and then serve.

Green Colada

Preparation Time: 5 minutes

Cooking time: 0 minute

Servings: 1

Ingredients:

1/2 cup frozen pineapple chunks

1/2 banana

1/2 teaspoon spirulina powder

1/4 teaspoon vanilla extract, unsweetened

1 cup of coconut milk

Directions:

Place all the Ingredients in the order in a food processor or blender and then pulse for 2 to 3 minutes at high speed until smooth. Pour the smoothie into a glass and then serve.

Berry Beet Velvet Smoothie

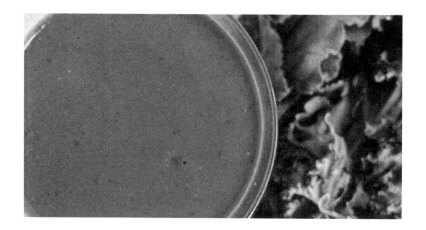

Preparation Time: 5 minutes

Cooking time: 0 minute

Servings: 1

Ingredients:

1/2 of frozen banana

1 cup mixed red berries

1 Medjool date, pitted

1 small beet, peeled, chopped

1 tablespoon cacao powder

1 teaspoon chia seeds

1/4 teaspoon vanilla extract, unsweetened

1/2 teaspoon lemon juice

2 teaspoons coconut butter

1 cup coconut milk, unsweetened

Directions:

Place all the Ingredients in the order in a food processor or blender and then pulse for 2 to 3 minutes at high speed until smooth. Pour the smoothie into a glass and then serve.

Strawberry, Banana and Coconut Shake

Preparation Time: 5 minutes

Cooking time: 0 minute

Servings: 1

Ingredients:

1 tablespoon coconut flakes

1 1/2 cups frozen banana slices

8 strawberries, sliced

1/2 cup coconut milk, unsweetened

1/4 cup strawberries for topping

Directions:

Place all the Ingredients in the order in a food processor or blender, except for topping and then pulse for 2 to 3 minutes at high speed until smooth. Pour the smoothie into a glass and then serve.

Ginger and Greens Smoothie

Preparation Time: 5 minutes

Cooking time: 0 minute

Servings: 1

Ingredients:

1 frozen banana

2 cups baby spinach

2-inch piece of ginger, peeled, chopped

¼ teaspoon cinnamon

¼ teaspoon vanilla extract, unsweetened

1/8 teaspoon salt

1 scoop vanilla protein powder

1/8 teaspoon cayenne pepper

2 tablespoons lemon juice

1 cup of orange juice

Directions:

Place all the Ingredients in the order in a food processor or blender and then pulse for 2 to 3 minutes at high speed until smooth. Pour the smoothie into a glass and then serve.

Chocolate Cherry Smoothie

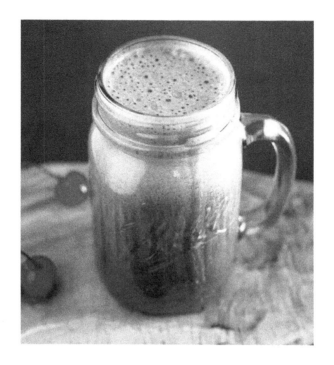

Preparation Time: 5 minutes

Cooking time: 0 minute

Servings: 1

Ingredients:

1 1/2 cups frozen cherries, pitted

1 cup spinach

1/2 small frozen banana

2 tablespoon cacao powder, unsweetened

1 tablespoon chia seeds

1 scoop of vanilla protein powder

1 teaspoon spirulina

1 1/2 cups almond milk, unsweetened

Directions:

Place all the Ingredients in the order in a food processor or blender and then pulse for 2 to 3 minutes at high speed until smooth. Pour the smoothie into a glass and then serve.

Kale and Spinach Smoothie

Preparation Time: 5 minutes

Cooking time: 0 minute

Servings: 1

Ingredients:

1 cup spinach

1 cup kale

1 frozen banana

3 small dates, pitted

1 1/4 cup almond milk, unsweetened

1 scoop of vanilla protein powder

1 teaspoon cinnamon

Directions:

Place all the Ingredients in the order in a food processor or blender and then pulse for 2 to 3 minutes at high speed until smooth. Pour the smoothie into a glass and then serve.

Peanut Butter and Coffee Smoothie

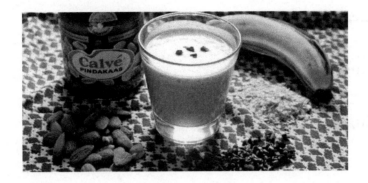

Preparation Time: 5 minutes

Cooking time: 0 minute

Servings: 1

Ingredients:

2 small frozen banana

1/2 teaspoon ground turmeric

1 tablespoon chia seeds

1 scoop of chocolate protein powder

2 tablespoons Peanut Butter

1 cup strong coffee, brewed

Directions:

Place all the Ingredients in the order in a food processor or blender and then pulse for 2 to 3 minutes at high speed until smooth. Pour the smoothie into a glass and then serve.

Broccoli and Quinoa Breakfast Patties

Preparation Time: 5 minutes

Cooking time: 6 minutes

Servings: 4

Ingredients:

1 cup cooked quinoa, cooked

1/2 cup shredded broccoli florets

1/2 cup shredded carrots

2 cloves of garlic, minced

2 teaspoon parsley

1 1/2 teaspoon onion powder

1 1/2 teaspoon garlic powder

1/3 teaspoon salt

1/4 teaspoon black pepper

1/2 cup bread crumbs, gluten-free

2 tablespoon coconut oil

2 flax eggs

Directions:

Prepare patties and for this, place all the Ingredients in a large bowl, except for oil and stir until well combined and then shape the mixture into patties. Take a skillet pan, place it over medium heat, add oil and when hot, add prepared patties in it and cook for 3 minutes per side until golden brown and crispy. Serve patties with vegan sour creams.

Sweet Potato Breakfast Hash

Preparation Time: 5 minutes

Cooking time: 28 minutes

Servings: 4

Ingredients:

4 cups cubed sweet potatoes, peeled

1/2 teaspoon sea salt

1/2 teaspoon turmeric

1/2 teaspoon cumin

1 teaspoon smoked paprika

2 cups diced white onion

2 cloves of garlic, peeled, minced

1/4 cup chopped cilantro

1 tablespoon coconut oil

½ cup vegan guacamole, for serving

1 ½ cup pica de Gallo

Directions:

Take a skillet pan, place it over medium heat, add oil and when it melts, add onion, potatoes, and garlic, season with salt, paprika, turmeric, and cumin, stir and cook for 25 minutes until potatoes are slightly caramelized. Then remove the pan from heat, add cilantro and distribute evenly between serving plates. Top the sweet potato hash with guacamole and pico de gallo and then serve.

Scrambled Eggs with Aquafaba

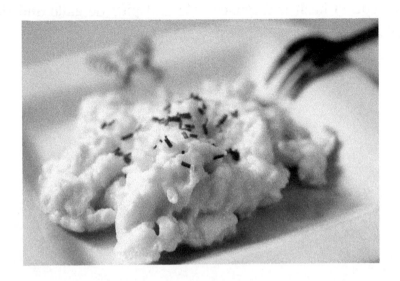

Preparation Time: 5 minutes

Cooking time: 15 minutes

Servings: 2

Ingredients:

6 ounces tofu, firm, pressed, drained

1/2 cup aquafaba

1 1/2 tablespoons olive oil

1 tablespoon nutritional yeast

1/4 teaspoon black salt

1/8 teaspoon ground turmeric

1/4 teaspoon ground black pepper

Directions:

Take a food processor, add tofu, yeast, black pepper, salt, and turmeric, then pour in aquafaba and olive oil and pulse for 1 minute until smooth. Take a skillet pan, place it over medium heat, and when hot, add tofu mixture and cook for 1 minute. Cover the pan, continue cooking for 3 minutes, then uncover the pan and pull the mixture across the pan with a wooden spoon until soft forms. Continue cooking for 10 minutes until resembles soft scrambled eggs, folding tofu mixture gently and heat over medium heat, then remove the pan from heat and season with salt and black pepper to taste. Serve straight away

Enchilada Breakfast Casserole

Preparation Time: 10 minutes

Cooking time: 25 minutes

Servings: 8

Ingredients:

15 ounces cooked corn

1 batch of vegan breakfast eggs

15 ounces cooked pinto beans

3 medium zucchini, sliced into rounds

10 ounces of vegan cheddar cheese, shredded

24 ounces red enchilada sauce

12 corn tortillas, cut into wedges Shredded lettuce for serving

Vegan sour cream for serving

Directions:

Take a skillet pan, grease it with oil and press the vegan breakfast eggs into the bottom of the pan in an even layer. Spread with 1/3 of enchilada sauce, then sprinkle with half of the cheese and cover with half of the tortilla wedges. Cover the wedges with 1/3 of the sauce, then layer with beans, corn, and zucchini, cover with remaining tortilla wedges, and spread the remaining sauce on top. Cover the pan with lid, place it over medium heat and cook for 25 minutes until cheese had melted, zucchini is tender, and sauce is bubbling. When done, let the casserole stand for 10 minutes, top with lettuce and sour cream, then cut the casserole into wedges, and serve.

Sweet Crepes

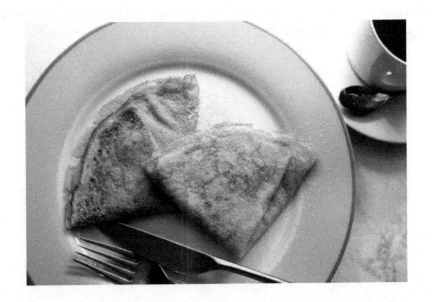

Preparation Time: 5 minutes

Cooking time: 8 minutes

Servings: 5

Ingredients:

1 cup of water

1 banana

1/2 cup oat flour

1/2 cup brown rice flour

1 teaspoon baking powder

1 tablespoon coconut sugar

1/8 teaspoon salt

Directions:

Take a blender, place all the Ingredients in it except for sugar and salt and pulse for 1 minute until smooth. Take a skillet pan, place it over medium-high heat, grease it with oil and when hot, pour in ¼ cup of batter, spread it as thin as possible, and cook for 2 to 3 minutes per side until golden brown. Cook remaining crepes in the same manner, then sprinkle with sugar and salt and serve

Tomato and Asparagus Quiche

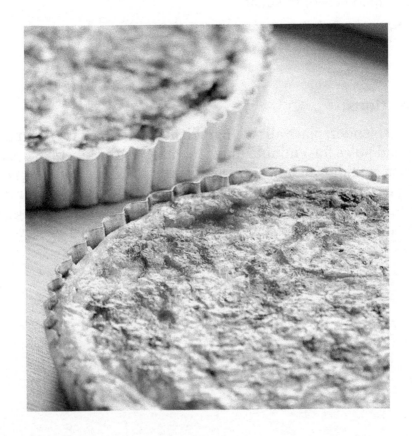

Preparation Time: 40 minutes

Cooking time: 35 minutes

Servings: 12

Ingredients:

For the Dough:

2 cups whole wheat flour

1/2 teaspoon salt

3/4 cup vegan margarine

1/3 cup water

For the Filling:

14 oz silken tofu

6 cherry tomatoes, halved

2 green onions, cut into rings

10 sun-dried tomatoes, in oil, chopped

7 oz green asparagus, diced

1 1/2 tablespoons herbs de Provence

1 tablespoon cornstarch

1 teaspoon turmeric

3 tablespoons olive oil

Directions:

Switch on the oven, then set it to 350 degrees F and let it preheat. Pre the dough and for this, take a bowl, place all the Ingredients for it, beat until incorporated, then knead for 5 minutes until smooth and refrigerate the dough for 30 minutes. Meanwhile, take a skillet pan, place it over medium heat, add 1 tablespoon oil and when hot, add green onion and cook for 2 minutes, set aside until required. Place a pot half full wit salty water over medium heat, bring it to boil, then add asparagus and boil for 3 minutes until tender, drain and set aside until required. Take a medium bowl, add tofu along with herbs de Provence, starch, turmeric,

47

and oil, whisk until smooth and then fold in tomatoes, green onion, and asparagus until mixed. Divide the prepared dough into twelve sections, take a muffin tray, line it twelve cups with baking cups, and then press a dough ball at the bottom of each cup and all the way up. Fill the cups with prepared tofu mixture, top with tomatoes, and bake for 35 minutes until cooked. Serve straight away.

Ultimate Breakfast Sandwich

Preparation Time: 40 minutes

Cooking time: 10 minutes

Servings: 4

Ingredients:

For the Tofu:

12 ounces tofu, extra-firm, pressed, drain

1/2 teaspoon garlic powder

1 teaspoon liquid smoke

2 tablespoons nutritional yeast

1 teaspoon Sriracha sauce

2 tablespoons soy sauce

2 tablespoons olive oil

2 tablespoons water

For the Vegan Breakfast Sandwich:

1 large tomato, sliced

4 English muffins, halved, toasted

1 avocado, mashed

Directions:

Prepare tofu, and for this, cut tofu into four slices and set aside. Stir together remaining Ingredients of tofu, pour the mixture into a bag, then add tofu pieces, toss until coated and marinate for 30 minutes. Take a skillet pan, place it over medium-high heat, add tofu slices along with the marinade and cook for 5 minutes per side. Prepare sandwich and for this, spread mashed avocado on the inner of the muffin, top with a slice of tofu, layer with a tomato slice and then serve.

Pancake

Preparation Time: 10 minutes

Cooking time: 18 minutes

Servings: 4

Ingredients:

Dry Ingredients:

1 cup buckwheat flour

1/8 teaspoon salt

½ teaspoon gluten-free baking powder

½ teaspoon baking soda

Wet Ingredients:

1 tablespoon almond butter

2 tablespoon maple syrup

1 tablespoon lime juice

1 cup coconut milk, unsweetened

Directions:

Take a medium bowl, add all the dry Ingredients and stir until mixed. Take another bowl, place all the wet Ingredients, whisk until combined, and then gradually whisk in dry Ingredients mixture until smooth and incorporated. Take a frying pan, place it over medium heat, add 2 teaspoons oil and when hot, drop in batter and cook for 3 minutes per side until cooked and lightly browned. Serve pancakes and fruits and maple syrup.

Herb & Cheese Omelet

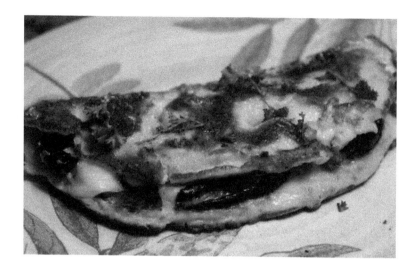

Preparation Time: 5 minutes

Cooking time: 5 minutes

Servings: 2

Ingredients:

4 eggs

Salt and pepper to taste

2 tbsp. low-fat milk

1 tsp. chives, chopped

1 tbsp. parsley, chopped

½ cup goat cheese, crumbled

1 tsp. olive oil

Directions:

Beat the eggs in a bowl. Stir in the salt, pepper and milk. In a bowl, combine the chives, parsley and goat cheese. Pour the oil into a pan over medium heat. Cook the eggs for 3 minutes. Add the cheese mixture on top. Fold and serve.

Green Breakfast Salad

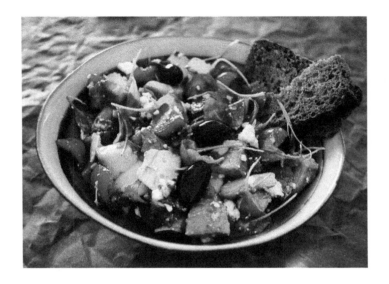

Preparation Time: 10 minutes

Cooking time: 10 minutes

Servings: 4

Ingredients:
1 tablespoon lemon juice
4 red bell peppers
1 lettuce head, cut into strips
Salt and black pepper to the taste
3 tablespoons coconut cream

2 tablespoons olive oil

1 ounces rocket leaves

Directions:

Place bell pepper in your air fryer's basket, cook at 400 degrees F for 10 minutes, transfer to a bowl, leave them aside to cool down, peel, cut them in strips and put them in a bowl. Add rocket leaves and lettuce strips and toss. In a bowl, mix oil with lemon juice, coconut cream, salt and pepper, whisk well, add over the salad, toss to coat, divide between plates and serve for breakfast. Enjoy!

Wheat Quick Bread

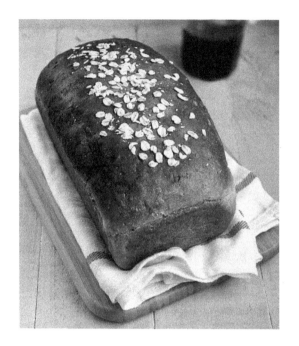

Servings: 1 loaf

Preparation Time: 10 mins

Cooking time: 20 mins

Ingredients:

1 cup rolled oats

1 cup whole wheat flour

1 cup soy milk

2 tsp. baking powder

1½ tbsp. agave syrup

1 tbsp. vegetable oil

1 tsp. salt

Directions:

Preheat the oven to 450 degrees Fahrenheit. In a food processor or blender, grind the oatmeal to make oatmeal flour. Combine oatmeal flour, whole wheat flour, baking powder and salt. In a separate bowl, dissolve the agave syrup in vegetable oil, and then stir in the soy milk. Combine both the dry and wet mixtures and stir until they form a soft dough. Form the dough into a smooth round ball and place on a lightly oiled baking sheet. Bake in for 20 minutes, or until the bottom crust of loaf sounds hollow when tapped.

Sweet Pomegranate Porridge

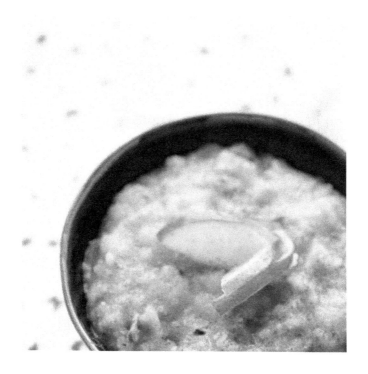

Preparation Time: 5 minutes

Cooking time: 30 minutes

Servings: 4

Ingredients:

2 Cups Oats

1 ½ Cups Water

1 ½ Cups Pomegranate Juice

2 Tablespoons Pomegranate Molasses

Directions:

Pour all Ingredients into the instant pot and mix well. Seal the lid, and cook on high pressure for four minutes. Use a quick release, and serve warm.

Potato and Zucchini Omelet

Preparation Time: 5 minutes

Cooking time: 20 minutes

Ingredients:

½ lb. potato (about 1¼ cups diced)

½ lb. zucchini (about 1½ cups diced)

⅔ cup chopped onion (1 small)

1 Tbs. butter

2 Tbs. olive oil

¼ tsp. dried dill weed

¼ tsp. dried basil, crushed

½ tsp. crushed dried red pepper

salt to taste

fresh-ground black pepper to taste

5 to 6 eggs

butter for frying

garnish sour cream

Directions:

Peel or scrub the potato and cut it in ½-inch dice. Wash, trim, and finely dice the zucchini. Drop the diced potato into boiling salted water and cook for 5 minutes, then drain it and set it aside.

Cook the diced zucchini in boiling water for 3 to 4 minutes, drain, and set aside. Heat the butter and the olive oil in a medium-sized skillet and sauté the onions in it until they start to color. Add the partially cooked potato and zucchini, the dill weed, basil, crushed red pepper, and salt. Cook this mixture over medium heat, stirring often, until the potatoes are just tender. Grind in some black pepper and add more salt if needed. Make either 2 medium-sized or 3 small omelets according to the directions. When the eggs are almost set, spoon some of the hot vegetables onto one side and fold the other side of the omelet over the filling. Slide the omelets out onto warm plates and serve immediately with sour cream.

Tomato Omelet

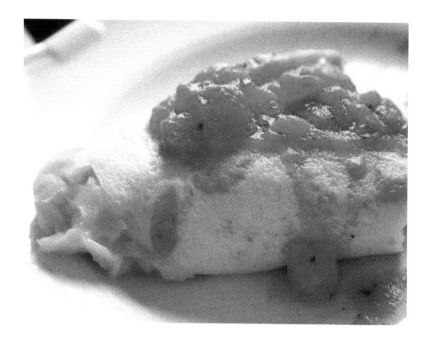

Preparation Time: 5 minutes

Cooking time: 40 minutes

Servings: 3

Ingredients:

8 medium sized tomatoes

2 cloves garlic 2 bay leaves

½ tsp. dried tarragon, crushed

1 tsp. salt, and more to taste

2 Tbs. chopped fresh parsley

1 medium-sized yellow onion

3 Tbs. olive oil

½ tsp. dried basil, crushed

5 cured black olives, pitted and sliced

coarse ground

black pepper to taste

8 to 10 eggs

Milk

Directions:

Blanch the tomatoes in boiling water for about 2 minutes and then peel them. Chop the tomatoes very coarsely and put them aside in a bowl with the salt. Chop the onion, mince the garlic, and sauté them in the olive oil in a large skillet until they begin to show color. Add the bay leaves and sauté a few minutes more. Add the tomatoes, the basil, tarragon, parsley, and sliced olives, and cook over medium heat, stirring occasionally, until the sauce is thick. It should take about 40 to 45 minutes. Make individual omelets according to the directions. Spoon on some of the hot Provençale sauce just when the eggs are nearly set. Blanch the tomatoes in boiling water for about 2 minutes and then peel them. Chop the tomatoes very coarsely and put them aside in a bowl with the salt. Chop the onion, mince the garlic, and sauté them in the olive oil in a large skillet until they begin to show color. Add the bay leaves and sauté a few minutes more. Add the tomatoes, the basil, tarragon, parsley, and sliced olives, and cook over medium heat, stirring occasionally, until the sauce is thick. It should take about 40 to 45 minutes. Make individual omelets according to the directions. Spoon on some of the hot Provençale sauce just when the eggs are nearly set, and fold the omelets over the sauce. Serve.

Vegan Tropical Pina Colada Smoothie

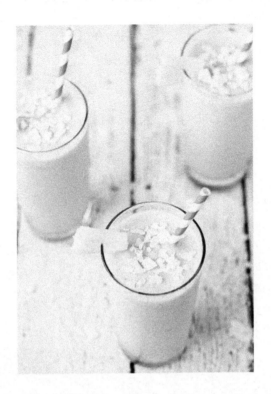

Preparation Time: 5 minutes

Cooking time: 0 minutes

1 smoothie.

Ingredients:

¾ cup soymilk

½ cup coconut milk

1 banana 1 ½ tbsp.

ground flax seed

1 tsp. vanilla

1 cup pineapple

1 tbsp. agave nectar

3 ice cubes

Directions:

Bring all the above Ingredients together in a blender, and blend the Ingredients to achieve your desired smoothie consistency. Enjoy!

Peach Protein Bars

Servings: 6

Preparation Time: 60 min

Ingredients:

1 cup flax seeds

½ cup peanuts

¼ cup hemp seeds

15g dehydrated peaches

2 tbsp. psyllium husk

¼ tsp. stevia

½ tsp. salt

1¼ cup water

Total number of Ingredients: 8

Directions:

Preheat oven at 350°F. Grind up nuts and seeds with ½ cup water in a blender, but make sure the mixture is not finely ground. Transfer and combine mixture with psyllium husk and cinnamon in a mixing bowl. Crush the dehydrated peaches into small bits and add to mixing bowl. Stir in the remaining water and salt until all Ingredients are combined. Let the mixture sit for a few minutes. Spread the mixture out on a baking sheet lined with parchment paper, and make sure the dough is about ¼ inch thick.

Bake for 45 minutes, remove around 30 minutes to cut the dough carefully in six pieces, and bake for another 15 minutes. Remove from oven and cool for 30 minutes. Can be stored for a week or frozen up to two months.

Breakfast Tacos

Preparation Time: 10 minutes

Cooking time: 6 minutes

Servings: 4

Ingredients

½ cup grape tomatoes, quartered

1 avocado, sliced

8 corn tortillas

Freshly ground black pepper

¼ teaspoon salt

¼ teaspoon cumin

¼ teaspoon ground turmeric

1 package firm tofu

1 garlic clove, minced

1 red pepper, diced

1 teaspoon olive oil

Directions:

Heat oil in a skillet over medium heat. Add in garlic and red pepper and sauté for around 2 minutes. Using your hands, crumble the tofu and add into the pan; and then add the seasonings. Cook for around 5 minutes making sure that you stir frequently. Taste and adjust the seasonings then apportion it and store in containers for the week. When you want to serve, simply put the scramble on tortillas, add any other toppings and enjoy.

Breakfast Cookies

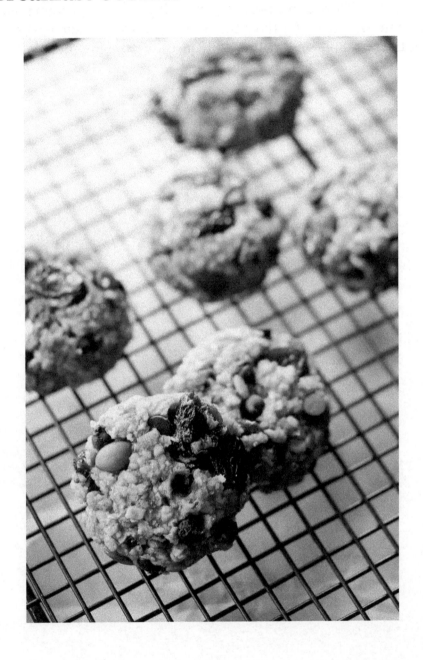

Preparation Time: 10 minutes

Cooking time: 6 minutes

Makes 24-32

Ingredients

Dry Ingredients

½ teaspoon baking powder

2 cups rolled oats

½ teaspoon baking soda

Wet Ingredients

1 teaspoon pure vanilla extract

2 flax eggs (2 tablespoons ground flaxseed and around 6 tablespoons of water, mix and put aside for 15 minutes)

2 tablespoons melted coconut oil

2 tablespoons pure maple syrup

½ cup natural creamy peanut butter

2 ripe bananas

Add-in Ingredients

½ cup finely chopped walnuts

½ cup raisins

Optional Topping

2 tablespoons chopped walnuts

2 tablespoons raisins

73

Directions:

Preheat the oven to 325 degrees F, and then use parchment paper to line a baking sheet and put aside. Add the bananas in a large bowl, and then use a fork to mash them until smooth. Add in the other wet Ingredients and mix until well incorporated. Add the dry Ingredients and then use a rubber spatula to stir and fold them into the dry Ingredients until well mixed. Stir in the walnuts and raisins. Scoop the cookie dough onto the prepared baking sheet making sure that you leave adequate space between the cookies. Bake in the preheated oven for around 12 minutes. Once ready, let the cookies cool on the baking sheet for around 10 minutes. Lift the cookies carefully from the baking sheet onto a cooling rack to further cool. Store the cookies in an airtight container in the fridge or at room temperature for up to one week.

Quick Breakfast Yogurt

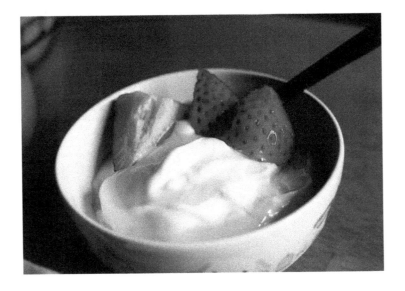

Preparation Time: 2 minutes

Cooking time: 8 min

Servings: 6

Ingredients:

4 cups Full-Fat Coconut Milk

2 tbsp Coconut Milk Powder

100 grams Strawberries, for serving

Directions:

Whisk together coconut milk and milk powder in a microwave safe bowl. Heat on high for 8-9 minutes. Top with fresh strawberries and choice of sweetener to serve.

Keto Breakfast Porridge

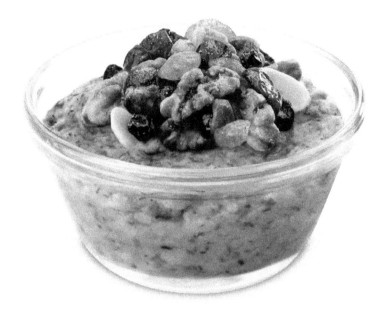

Preparation Time: 5 minutes

Cooking time: 5 minutes

Servings: 4

Ingredients:
1 cup Flaked Coconut
½ cup Hemp Seeds
1 tbsp Coconut Flour
1 cup Water

½ cup Coconut Cream

1 tbsp Ground Cinnamon

1 tbsp Erythritol

Directions:

Combine all Ingredients in a pot. Simmer for 5 minutes, stirring continuously.

Scrambled Tofu

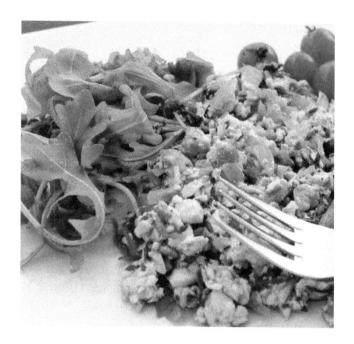

Preparation Time: 10 minutes

Cooking time: 30 minutes

Servings: 4

Ingredients:

2 tablespoons coconut aminos

1 block firm tofu, cubed

1 teaspoon turmeric powder

2 tablespoons olive oil

½ teaspoon onion powder

½ teaspoon garlic powder

2 and ½ cup red potatoes, cubed

½ cup yellow onion, chopped

Salt and black pepper to the taste

Directions:

In a bowl, mix tofu with 1 tablespoon oil, salt, pepper, coconut aminos, garlic and onion powder, turmeric and onion and toss to coat. In another bowl, mix potatoes with the rest of the oil, salt and pepper and toss. Put potatoes in preheated air fryer at 350 degrees F and bake for 15 minutes, shaking them halfway Add tofu and the marinade and bake at 350 degrees F for 15 minutes. Divide between plates and serve. Enjoy!

Breakfast Polenta

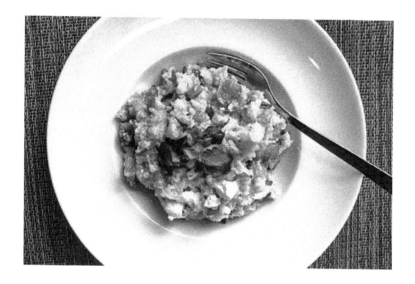

Preparation Time: 10 minutes

Cooking time: 15 minutes

Servings: 4

Ingredients:

1 cup cornmeal

3 cups water

Cooking spray

1 tablespoon coconut oil

Maple syrup for serving

Directions:

Put the water for the polenta in a pot and heat up over medium heat. Add cornmeal, stir well and cook for 10 minutes. Add oil, stir again, cook for 2 minutes more, take off heat, leave aside to cool down, take spoon fools of polenta, shape balls and place them on a lined baking sheet. Grease your air fryer basket with the cooking spray , place polenta balls inside and cook them for 16 minutes at 380 degrees F flipping them halfway. Divide polenta balls between plates and serve them with some maple syrup on top. Enjoy!

Breakfast Muffins

Preparation Time: 10 minutes

Cooking time: 6 minutes

Servings: 4

Ingredients

2 cups diced banana

½ cup coconut milk, unsweetened

¼ cup coconut oil, melted

1 cup frozen sliced strawberries

2 teaspoons maple syrup

1 tablespoon ground flaxseed

⅓ cup almond flour

½ cup dates

Directions:

Line muffin tins and set aside. Then add ground flax seeds, almond meal and dates into a food processor. Pulse the mixture until it becomes crumbly and then transfer to a bowl. At this point, stir in maple syrup and then press a tablespoon of crust mixture into the bottom of the muffin gently, to make the crust. Put semi-thawed strawberries in a food processor and pulse until smooth. Add in coconut and coconut milk slowly until you achieve a thick, sorbet consistency. In a bowl, add in the strawberries and gently fold in the bananas. Then sub-divide the strawberry banana mixture over the top of the crust evenly. Finally put the muffins in a freezer and let it freeze and solidify. Once frozen place in freezer bags and freeze. To serve, thaw for around 15 minutes and then serve

Bean Salsa Breakfast

Preparation Time: 10 minutes

Cooking time: 6 minutes

Servings: 2

Ingredients

Olive oil

½ lemon

1 avocado

2 cloves of garlic

2 handfuls of spinach

1 handful of basil

6 cherry tomatoes

4 spring onions

1 can of haricot beans

Black pepper

Himalayan salt

Directions:

Chop the onions and the garlic and then halve the cherry tomatoes. Let 50ml water to boil in a frying pan and then steam-fry the garlic for a few seconds. Throw in the spring onions, haricot beans and the cherry tomatoes and cook until soft. Now add in the spinach and basil and cook until wilted, and season with the black pepper and Himalayan salt. Meanwhile, halve the avocado. To serve, top the bean mixture with halved avocado and lemon. You can drizzle olive oil all over the dish. Alternatively, you can freeze the bean mixture for another day. When serving, top with an avocado and some lemon.

Gingerbread-Spiced Breakfast Smoothie

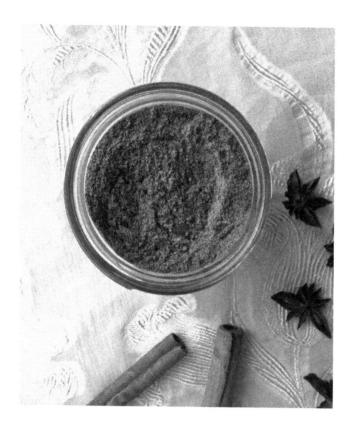

Preparation Time: 2 minutes

Servings: 2

Ingredients:

1 cup Coconut Milk

1 bag Tea

¼ tsp Cinnamon Powder

1/8 tsp Nutmeg Powder

1/8 tsp Powdered Cloves

1/3 cup Chia Seeds

2 tbsp Flax Seeds

Directions:

Put the teabag in a mug and pour in a cup of hot water. Allow to steep for a few minutes. Pour the tea into a blender together with the rest of the Ingredients. Process until smooth.

Maca Caramel Frap

Preparation time: 5 minutes

Cooking time: 0 minute

Servings: 4

Ingredients:

1/2 of frozen banana, sliced

1/4 cup cashews, soaked for 4 hours

2 Medjool dates, pitted

1 teaspoon maca powder

1/8 teaspoon sea salt

1/2 teaspoon vanilla extract, unsweetened

1/4 cup almond milk, unsweetened

1/4 cup cold coffee, brewed

Directions:

Place all the ingredients in the order in a food processor or blender and then pulse for 2 to 3 minutes at high speed until smooth. Pour the smoothie into a glass and then serve.

Peach Crumble Shake

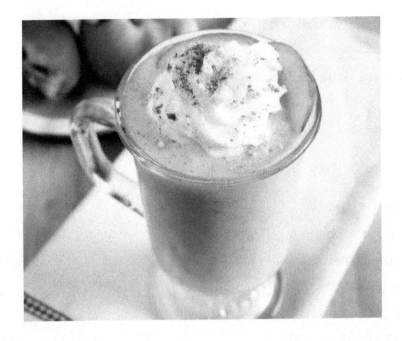

Preparation time: 5 minutes

Cooking time: 0 minute

Servings: 1

Ingredients:

1 tablespoon chia seeds

¼ cup rolled oats

2 peaches, pitted, sliced

¾ teaspoon ground cinnamon

1 Medjool date, pitted

½ teaspoon vanilla extract, unsweetened

2 tablespoons lemon juice

½ cup of water

1 tablespoon coconut butter

1 cup coconut milk, unsweetened

Directions:

Place all the ingredients in the order in a food processor or blender and then pulse for 2 to 3 minutes at high speed until smooth. Pour the smoothie into a glass and then serve.

Banana Bread Shake With Walnut Milk

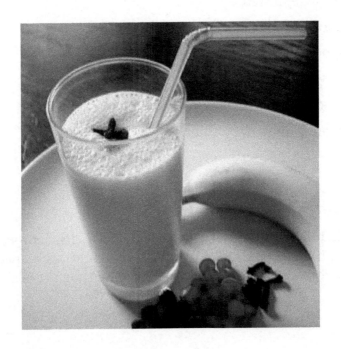

Preparation time: 5 minutes

Cooking time: 0 minute

Servings: 2

Ingredients:

2 cups sliced frozen bananas

3 cups walnut milk

1/8 teaspoon grated nutmeg

1 tablespoon maple syrup

1 teaspoon ground cinnamon

1/2 teaspoon vanilla extract, unsweetened

2 tablespoons cacao nibs

Directions:

Place all the ingredients in the order in a food processor or blender and then pulse for 2 to 3 minutes at high speed until smooth. Pour the smoothie into two glasses and then serve.

Peanut Butter and Mocha Smoothie

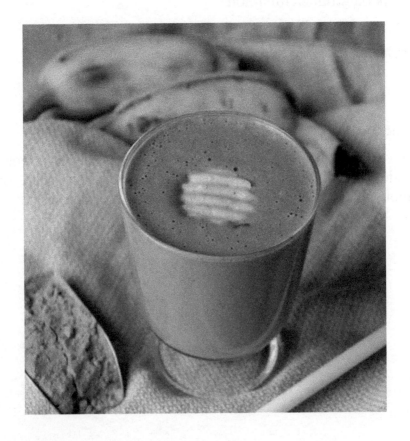

Preparation time: 5 minutes

Cooking time: 0 minute

Servings: 1

Ingredients:

1 frozen banana, chopped

1 scoop of chocolate protein powder

2 tablespoons rolled oats

1/8 teaspoon sea salt

¼ teaspoon vanilla extract, unsweetened

1 teaspoon cocoa powder, unsweetened

2 tablespoons peanut butter

1 shot of espresso

½ cup almond milk, unsweetened

Directions:

Place all the ingredients in the order in a food processor or blender and then pulse for 2 to 3 minutes at high speed until smooth. Pour the smoothie into a glass and then serve.

Sweet Potato Smoothie

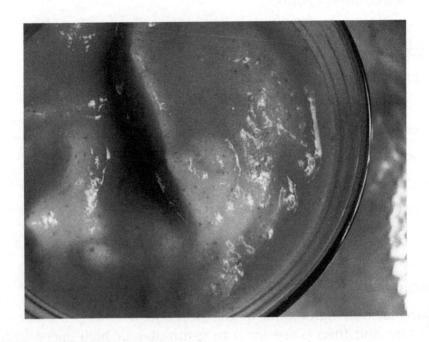

Preparation time: 5 minutes

Cooking time: 0 minute

Servings: 1

Ingredients:

1/2 cup frozen zucchini pieces

1 cup cubed cooked sweet potato, frozen

1/2 frozen banana

1/2 teaspoon sea salt

1/2 teaspoon cinnamon

1 scoop of vanilla protein powder

1/4 teaspoon nutmeg

1 tablespoon almond butter

1 1/2 cups almond milk, unsweetened

Directions:

Place all the ingredients in the order in a food processor or blender and then pulse for 2 to 3 minutes at high speed until smooth. Pour the smoothie into a glass and then serve.

Lemon and Blueberry Smoothie

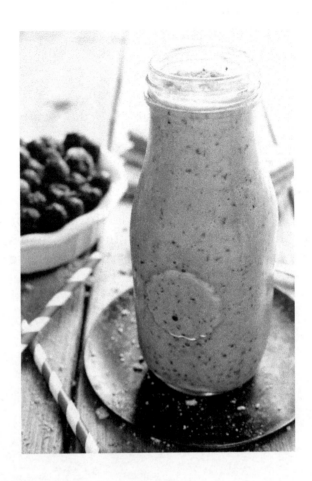

Preparation time: 5 minutes

Cooking time: 0 minute

Servings: 1

Ingredients:

1 1/2 cups frozen blueberries

1/2 frozen banana

1 tablespoon chia seeds

3 tablespoon lemon juice

1 teaspoon lemon zest

1 1/2 teaspoon cinnamon

1 1/2 cups almond milk, unsweetened

1 scoop of vanilla protein powder

Directions:

Place all the ingredients in the order in a food processor or blender and then pulse for 2 to 3 minutes at high speed until smooth. Pour the smoothie into a glass and then serve.

Beet and Orange Smoothie

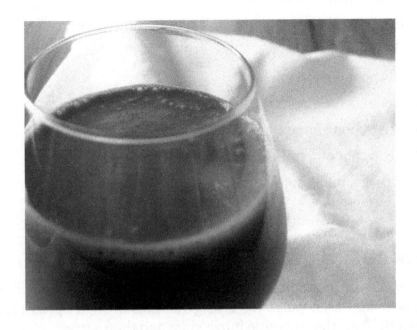

Preparation time: 5 minutes

Cooking time: 0 minute

Servings: 1

Ingredients:
1 cup chopped zucchini rounds, frozen
1 cup spinach
1 small peeled navel orange, frozen

1 small chopped beet

1 scoop of vanilla protein powder

1 cup almond milk, unsweetened

Directions:

Place all the ingredients in the order in a food processor or blender and then pulse for 2 to 3 minutes at high speed until smooth. Pour the smoothie into a glass and then serve

Chocolate, Avocado, and Banana Smoothie

Preparation time: 5 minutes

Cooking time: 0 minute

Servings: 1

Ingredients:

1 medium frozen banana

2 small dates, pitted

1/2 cup steamed and frozen cauliflower florets

1/4 of a medium avocado

1 teaspoon cinnamon

1 tablespoon cacao powder

1/2 teaspoon sea salt

1 teaspoon maca

1/2 scoop of vanilla protein powder

2 tablespoon cacao nibs

1 tablespoon almond butter

1 cup almond milk

Directions:

Place all the ingredients in the order in a food processor or blender and then pulse for 2 to 3 minutes at high speed until smooth. Pour the smoothie into a glass and then serve.

Scrambled Tofu Breakfast Tacos

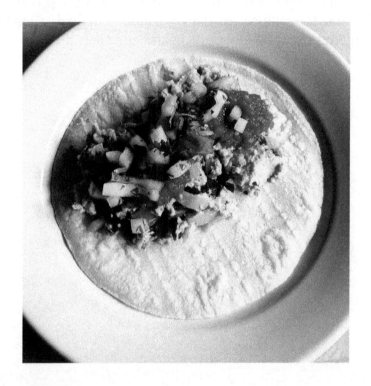

Preparation time: 5 minutes

Cooking time: 10 minutes

Servings: 4

Ingredients:

12 ounces tofu, pressed, drained

1/2 cup grape tomatoes, quartered

1 medium red pepper, diced

1 medium avocado, sliced

1 clove of garlic, minced

1/4 teaspoon ground turmeric

1/4 teaspoon ground black pepper

1/4 teaspoon salt

1/4 teaspoon cumin

1 teaspoon olive oil

8 corn tortillas

Directions:

Take a skillet pan, place it over medium heat, add oil and when hot, add pepper and garlic and cook for 2 minutes. Then add tofu, crumble it, sprinkle with black pepper, salt, and all the spices, stir and cook for 5 minutes. When done, distribute tofu between tortilla, top with tomato and avocado, and serve.

Chocolate Chip, Strawberry and Oat Waffles

Preparation time: 10 minutes

Cooking time: 25 minutes

Servings: 6

Ingredients:

6 tablespoons chocolate chips, semi-sweet

½ cup chopped strawberries

Powdered sugar as needed for topping

Dry

1/4 cup oats

1 1/2 tablespoon ground flaxseeds

1 1/2 cup whole wheat pastry flour

2 1/2 tablespoon cocoa powder

1/4 teaspoon salt

2 teaspoons baking powder

Wet Ingredients:

1/3 cup mashed bananas

2 tablespoon maple syrup

2 tablespoon coconut oil

1/2 teaspoon vanilla extract, unsweetened

1/4 cup applesauce, unsweetened

1 3/4 cup almond milk, unsweetened

Directions:

Take a medium bowl, place all the dry ingredients in it, and whisk until mixed. Take a large bowl, place all the wet ingredients in it, whisk until combined, and then whisk in dry ingredients mixture in four batches until incorporated, don't overmix. Let the batter stand at room temperature for 5 minutes and in the meantime, switch on the waffle iron and let it preheat until hot. Then ladle one-sixth of the batter in it and cook until golden brown and firm. Cook remaining waffles in the same manner and when done, top them with chocolate chips and berries, sprinkle with sugar and then serve

Lightning Source UK Ltd.
Milton Keynes UK
UKHW020704130521
383649UK00005B/113

9 781802 693614